Ketogenic Diet

The Ultimate Book For The Ketogenic Diet. Lose The Weight and Belly Fat FAST!

By

Martha Blake

Disclaimer

THIS BOOK IS NOT INTENDED TO BE A SUBSTITUTE FOR CONSULTAION WITH A PROFESSIONAL HEALTHCARE PRACTITIONER. PLEASE ALWAYS CONSULT WITH YOUR HEALTHCARE PRACTITIONER BEFORE STARTING ANY SUPPLEMENT OR DIET. THE PUBLISHER AND AUTHORS DISCLAIM ANY RESPONSILITY FOR ANY ADVERSE EFFFECTS REUSLT DIRECTLY OF INDIRECTLY FROM THE INFORMAITON CONTAINED IN THIS BOOK

Contents

Introduction

Fad diets are dime a dozen, and it can always be tempting to follow them. The promise of losing weight quickly is usually a hard one to resist. But many fad diets don't have a well-researched scientific basis. In the long run, they can do more harm than good.

Ketogenics, which has long been used as one of the ways to control epileptic seizures, has found new fame as a weight loss tool. There are sound reasons to consider this diet, but the most important tool before you make what will be a drastic lifestyle change is information. Instead of following a fad, where your health is concerned, you must make an informed choice.

So we will give you a rundown of what a ketogenic diet is, why it's considered a guaranteed way to lose weight, and all the factors you need to consider before you decide to go on a ketogenic diet. Bonus: personal observations of what worked and what didn't, and what was easiest to stick with.

After arming yourself with all the information, the next step is knowing how to do it – meal plans and recipes. This is a one stop resource to get your started on both the theory and the practical aspects of being on a ketogenic diet. Of course, remember that everybody is unique. Yours is, too. So before you start any diet, you should consult a doctor and get all the information you can about your own health, as well. It's an important part of being informed.

So now, start reading, and make sure that you make the decision that is right for you.

Ketogenic History

In common parlance, a ketogenic diet is one where your consumption of carbohydrates is extremely low. The purpose of a diet like this is to make sure your body, instead of burning carbohydrates for energy, has no choice but to burn fat for energy.

The purpose of a ketogenic diet is to make your body go into 'ketosis', where instead of burning glucose for energy, it burns ketones. Under normal circumstances and with most diets that we follow with a reasonable amount of carbohydrates, the carbs are our main source of energy. Carbohydrates are converted into glucose. But if you reduce your intake of carbohydrates drastically, the liver converts fatty acids to ketones, which are used for energy instead. Ketones can be used by the brain, the heart and different muscles for energy.

Originally, this diet was used to control epilepsy in children. For this purpose, their diets are modified to be high in fat, but low in protein and carbohydrates. Protein intake is limited to just what was necessary to maintain muscle development and the right weight according to height. This classic ketogenic diet sticks to a fat to combined protein and carbohydrates ratio of 4:1. To achieve this, intake of regular food like bread, pasta, rice, starchy vegetables, starchy fruits, grain-based foods and so on are drastically limited. Calorie consumption is mainly through fatty foods like butter, nuts, cream etc.

This method of controlling epilepsy was popular in the 1920s, though it wasn't understood why it helped control it. Popular advertisements claimed that fasting could cure, or at least control, epilepsy. Doctors claimed outrageous rates of success – some claiming that 90 percent of their paediatric patients were cured, which was later proven false – but hidden in their tall claims was data that proved that they did have a significant degree of success; just not as significant as they claimed. Some doctors, after a period of fasting, put their patients on long-term diets with very low starch and sugar, which helped them control their conditions with a fairly high rate of success.

As it was studied further, the link between low carbohydrate intake and production of ketones was discovered. Other effects of the ketogenic diet were also explored, and it was discovered that children on the ketogenic diet had better sleep, became more alert and behaved better, but often had problems with nausea because of the significant reduction of carbohydrates.

But in the decade after that, anti-convulsant medication became more prevalent and popular. That led to the fall in popularity of the ketogenic diet, until in the 1990s, when Jim Abrahams, a Hollywood producer, turned to the diet to keep his son's epilepsy under check. He established the Charlie Foundation, and this led to a second rise in popularity of the ketogenic diet. The publicity also made this a viable area of scientific research, and other potential benefits of the ketogenic diet began to be explored. This is how the potential use of a less strict and milder form of the ketogenic diet for weight loss was discovered, and came to become a mainstream method. More research was done, and it was discovered that MCTs – medium-chain triglycerides – can give more ketones than the more common kinds of dietary fats.

Even if you only heard of the ketogenic diet recently, you're bound to have known another diet that was very popular and based on similar principles: the Atkins diet. It's not as dramatically low in carbohydrates as the strictly ketogenic diet, but it does have the same basic idea. Most ketogenic meal plans you would follow at home share many similarities with the Atkins diet. The original Atkins diet book, published in 1972, made claims that haven't been backed up by later research, but many of the believed disadvantages of following it have been proven wrong in the 2000s. The Atkins diet has several stages, and the first stage is considered to be a fairly strict ketogenic diet.

The idea that making the body use fat as a primary energy source could help you both detox and lose weight gained traction in the 2000s. Low carbohydrate diets have become extremely popular, and there are multiple kinds to choose from. For instance, importance of the glycemic index is beginning to be recognised. This index measures how certain foods affect our blood sugar level – how steeply it rises after consumption of a specific food. This is one of the ways used to get an understanding of how carbohydrates are broken down and converted into energy by the body. A low glycemic index diet (Low GI diet) includes specific carbohydrates that are broken down more slowly by the body, keeping the blood sugar level more stable, rather than the steep highs and lows caused by, say, a candy bar.

So before you decide to embark on a ketogenic diet, you have to understand the basics of a low-carbohydrate diet and the variations thereof. This will help you make an informed decision as to whether a strict ketogenic diet or a more liberal low-carbohydrate diet would be more suited to your purpose.

How does the ketogenic diet work?

We've already covered the basic and most important part of the ketogenic diet: making the body go into the state called ketosis. This is accomplished by reducing carbohydrate intake to a degree that makes the liver break fatty acids down into ketones, that will give the body energy. Ketones take the place of glucose, which you get from the breaking down of carbohydrates and gives you energy.

But this begs the obvious question: how does getting your energy from ketones instead of glucose help you detox or lose weight?

First, not all the weight you lose will be fat. Ketosis is caused within the body by the increase of three biochemicals in your bloodstream: acetoacetic acid, acetone, and beta-hydroxybutyric acid. This increase will affect your body in many ways, and one of those ways is an attempt on your body's part to reduce the levels of sodium in your body. This means increased urination, which, in turn, means that you will lose quite a bit of water weight. One of the problems of the earlier forms of the ketogenic diet was the occurrence of kidney stones. This was caused because that form of fasting included the restriction of fluids at a time when the body needed more fluids than usual.

Second, while you will be consuming fewer carbohydrate- heavy foods, and more protein and fat, not all the energy will come from the food you eat. A lot of it will be through the breaking down of fatty acids in your body, which means, in simplistic terms, you will be burning fat.

Another reported effect of the ketogenic diet that is being explored in greater detail is that it will make you less hungry. The reduction of carbohydrates in your food will result in the suppression of appetite, which, naturally, means that you will eat less. All those empty calories caused by munching between meals because you feel peckish can be cut out.

This effect is also linked to how the insulin levels rise and fall. Think of how you feel when you have a candy bar. You feel low before you have it, but you get an instant spike in energy as soon as you do. But you know that it won't last. You will be hyperactive and a bit jumpy for a while, and then you can feel your blood sugar dipping. This will make your body crave more energy, and you reach for another candy bar or a high carbohydrate food that will give you that spike again. Starchy and sugary foods can have this effect. To keep this craving at bay, you have to keep your sugar levels steady, and the foods that you're encouraged to eat on a ketogenic diet can help with this.

However, a very important thing to remember is that your weight loss will still be linked to how many calories you consume. If you consume more calories than you use up, you will still gain weight. But if you control your calorie consumption and reduce your carbohydrate consumption as well, your body will be forced to burn the fat already stored in your body for energy. This will result not only in weight loss, but in the right kind of weight loss. As long as you ensure that you get enough protein, which is one of the major ways in which ketogenic diets for weight loss differs from the form of ketogenic diets used for controlling epilepsy, you can lose fat without sacrificing your muscle mass.

Controlling insulin levels is a very important factor that makes ketogenic diets work well. Low levels of blood glucose, if maintained, can urge the pancreas to start releasing glucagon. Glucagon, in turn, makes the liver turn to the reserves of stored glycogen, and convert it to glucose. This is released into the blood stream. Eventually, the glycogen reserves in your liver will be exhausted and there will be no more glucose for your body to find. This is when the body turns to fatty acids. The brain needs energy, but the brain cannot use energy in the form of fatty acids. So these fatty acids are converted into ketones, which serve as primary energy source for the brain. This is usually accompanied by gluconeogenesis, which is the conversion of protein to glucose. This ensures that your blood glucose levels will not fall too low to function well.

It is also important to distinguish between the fats you are encouraged to consume in ketogenic diets and the fats you usually end up consuming on a daily basis. Trans fats are strictly discouraged, and trans fats are the culprits most often linked to heart diseases and high cholesterol. Advocates of the ketogenic diet often point out that high insulin levels encourage the storage of fat, and this is one of the main reasons why high-fat diets are linked to so many health risks. If you counter that problem with a solution that involves controlling insulin levels, which is one of the cornerstones of the ketogenic diet, it is no longer the kind of risk we're used to associating with fats.

Ketoacidosis: Should you be worried?

If you have mentioned to anybody that you're considering the ketogenic diet, you will have got the obligatory warning: ketoacidosis. But there is a lot of misinformation surrounding this particular scary sounding word, so let's clear some of it up.

Let's get this out of the way first: ketoacidosis is a perfectly legitimate condition and one that can be very dangerous. When you start on a ketogenic diet, you should know that a mild form of acidosis is not out of the ordinary. That sounds frightening, but the scary bit is over. The rest of it is far more reassuring.

Ketogenic diets are not, by any stretch of numbers or the imagination, the primary cause of ketoacidosis. Ketoacidosis is primarily caused by untreated type I diabetes, though occasionally also type II diabetes, and alcoholism.

First, let's come to grips with what ketoacidosis is. It's a metabolic state induced by extreme and uncontrolled ketosis. Note the terms 'extreme' and 'uncontrolled', two words that should never be associated with any reputed or respected ketogenic diet recommendation. It is caused by a drastic increase in ketone production; so drastic that your body cannot control it, and the levels of keto acids are so out of control that your blood pH value decreases dangerously, finally reaching a level that can even be fatal in extreme cases.

For otherwise healthy individuals whose insulin production has not shown any irregularities, such extreme ketosis is virtually impossible unless they go on such an extremely low calorie diet that their bodies cannot cope with it. This is not the only kind of danger associated with extreme low calorie diets, of course.

If you are diabetic and undiagnosed, instead of maintaining a steady level of low insulin, your body faces a severe shortage of insulin. This causes the body to go into overdrive, with the liver converting too much fatty acids into acidic ketone bodies, making you go into an advanced state of ketosis that can result in ketoacidosis. This is usually accompanied by dehydration, which can further exacerbate the condition, and hyperglycemia.

Of course, even if you know that you're perfectly healthy and need have no fear of ketoacidosis, it can be difficult to put something like that out of your mind. Most people, when you tell them that you're going on a new diet that they wouldn't try, love to scare you. So here are the symptoms of ketoacidosis:

- Dehydration, excessive thirst despite drinking lots of fluids and excessive urination
- Extreme nausea and vomiting
- Tender abdomen
- Difficulty breathing leading to needing deep breaths like gasps
- Mental fogginess and confusion

Remember that mild nausea is an expected side effect of the ketogenic diet, so don't panic if you feel a bit sick. These are not signs and symptoms that can be easily overlooked. There is an odour associated with ketogenic diets because of the increased production of acetone. Bad breath is unfortunately unavoidable. But ketoacidosis is associated with an extremely fruity, sickly sweet odour about you.

If somebody tells you that you smell like pear drops and you're not using a perfume with pear extracts, it's time to go to the hospital. This is extremely relevant for everybody, not just people looking to go on an extreme ketogenic diet of some sort. Undiagnosed diabetics are the people most likely to suffer from ketoacidosis.

Other triggers that might result in ketoacidosis are:

- Drug and alcohol abuse
- Intense physical or emotional trauma and stress
- Certain surgical procedures

Advantages of the ketogenic diet

One of the biggest advantages of the ketogenic diet for weight loss is that studies have shown that you can cut down your calorie consumption quite drastically without feeling ravenously hungry all the time. According to a paper published by the American Society for Clinical Nutrition, "A 2-week carefully controlled inpatient study showed that a ketogenic diet was beneficial for the control of weight and blood glucose concentrations in diabetic patients. Cutting carbohydrate consumption to ≈20 g/d produced a spontaneous reduction in calories of ≈1000 kcal/d with little change in hunger, diet satisfaction, or energy levels."

The paper goes on to recommend, "A suggestion for extending the benefits of ketogenic weight-loss diets would be to alternate 1–3 wk of the PSMF with longer periods of the Heller plan." The Heller plan allows a more flexible regimen, since it includes a full balanced meal.

If you can curb your hunger, you can lose weight, but with a low-carbohydrate diet, you can lose weight faster, at least for the first six months that you're on it. For the first couple of weeks, weight loss can be quite drastic. A study published in the New England Journal of Medicine explicitly compared weight loss over six months between those on a low-fat diet and those on a low-carbohydrate diet. The results showed that those on the low-carbohydrate diet had significantly more weight loss as well as reduction in triglyceride levels.

But what about after those six months? That's where you have to be careful and get creative. A low-carb diet, without the right meal plans and recipes, can seem quite restrictive. Most of the food we get is full of sugar and starches. So while you can up your carbohydrates intake to a certain level after you have reached your goal weight, you still have to keep it within certain limits. If you go back to old ways after reaching your goal weight, it's inevitable that you will put on weight again. It's important to think of going the low-carb way as a lifestyle change. Include treat days if you need to, but make sure that you keep a check on your eating habits.

One specification most people have about weight loss is that they want to lose it from their bellies. But everybody will tell you that spot reduction like that isn't possible. You can tone up specific parts of your body, and you can lose weight overall, but you can't lose weight only from a certain part, can you?

According to a paper published by Nutrition and Metabolism, you can. The study compared weight and fat loss as well as far loss specifically from the 'trunk' – basically the midsection – and found that even taking into account the increased overall fat loss, those on a very low carbohydrate diet lost comparatively more fat from their trunks.

One of the scare points brought up by people who don't want you to go on the ketogenic diet will be that your triglycerides will shoot up. This is a risk factor for many ailments, including heart disease. You might expect your triglycerides to shoot up, but, counter-intuitively, they go down. The study that compared subjects on a low-fat and a low-carb diet also made this observation.

Going on the ketogenic diet also inevitably means no sugar. Starch gets broken down into sugar, and you will be avoiding starches, so no indirect sugar, either. Avoiding these danger foods means that it is much easier for people, even those with type II diabetes, to control their blood sugar levels and insulin levels with a low-carbohydrate diet. This has helped people who have built up insulin resistance to live a far more productive life.

There are also some studies that suggest that the ketogenic diet can improve your good cholesterol levels and help you control high blood pressure, though these studies focused on specific groups of people. There are even suggestions that it can help stabilise thyroid conditions.

Even more promising, there are studies that suggest that the ketogenic diet can help prevent cancer. Research is being done into the theory that cancer cells predominantly use glucose for energy, and that there might be ways to link cancer with metabolic diseases. If this research is backed up over next few years with more affirmative studies, it might turn out that the ketogenic diet is an excellent way for those predisposed to cancer to stay a step ahead of the horrible condition. With more research, we'll have more information on which to base decisions regarding the ketogenic diet for better health.

The ketogenic diet changes the energy on which the brain functions. This could have long-term implications for the health of your brain cells, and so far, research shows that the results are favourable. Currently, research is being done to try to find out how the ketogenic diet could help people with Alzheimer's. Even in the 1920s, it was discovered that children on the ketogenic diet to control epilepsy were more alert. New studies, including one published in 2012 in Neurobiology of Aging, suggest that mild cognitive impairment can be stalled, and sometimes even reversed, with this diet.

This study concluded that they found "improved memory function with a medium effect size in individuals with Mild Cognitive Impairment in response to a relatively brief period of carbohydrate restriction designed to reduce insulin levels and induce ketone metabolism. To our knowledge, these data demonstrate for the first time that carbohydrate restriction can produce memory enhancement in this at-risk population."

Still more encouraging, studies are also being undertaken to find out if this diet can have a positive impact on neurodegenerative diseases like Parkinsons Disease or ALS. The results so far have been positive. There have even been studies linking the ketogenic diet with improvement in children with autism.

Disadvantages of the Ketogenic Diet

You might have got the impression that the ketogenic diet can solve just about every kind of worrying problem you've got. That isn't true. It's not a miracle diet. It is a tool that can be used to successfully control many conditions without depending too much on long-term prescription medicines, but there are disadvantages, too.

The first disadvantage you will notice is that you're not feeling very comfortable. You will feel nauseated quite often because your body does go into ketosis. It is not a comfortable thing to endure when your body has been used to getting sugar and starch as it pleases.

You will also notice that your breath gets worse. You could try chewing mints, but remember that sugar isn't allowed when you pick your gum. Acetone is a compound that will make your breath smell worse, and acetone is one of the acids that increase in your blood stream.

Another problem you might encounter is the very unpleasant one of constipation. This can be countered by making sure that you include lots of green, leafy vegetables in your diet. These vegetables are high in fibre and low in carbohydrates, so they will nourish you and keep your bowels from complaining too much.

Dehydration is another problem. You will need to consume a lot more fluid when you're on the ketogenic diet because your kidneys will be functioning overtime. If you don't compensate, remember that kidney stones are a realistic problem.

The problems that you will have to deal with include general discomfort: headaches, nausea, slight dizziness, trouble sleeping, muscle aches and a lingering thirst. Remember to refer to the symptoms of ketoacidosis. Even if you're at very little risk of developing this, especially since most ketogenic diets for weight loss will include enough protein and vegetables, you should know where to draw the line between being mildly uncomfortable and feeling sick enough to need attention.

Ingredients to Work with

If you have gone through all those details and decided that you do want to go on the ketogenic diet, good work. It means you are dedicated and goal-oriented, and there is a good chance that you can manage to keep it off once you take it off.

It takes a little time to get used to cooking on a ketogenic diet. Most of the interesting meals we make have grains, flour or starchy vegetables in them. It can be daunting. But the very fact that you have made the choice to go on this diet shows that you are brave enough to venture into a new kind of cuisine. There are excellent ways to make ketogenic meals interesting.

First, come to grips with the ingredients you may use and how you may use them.

Fats:

You will be having more fats than usual when you're on the ketogenic diet, but you have to be sure you're having the right kinds of fats. You want to avoid trans fats as far as possible, so focus on good fats, like olive oil, coconut oil, butter, avocados and so on. You can use vegetable oils, but try to restrict yourself to 'cold-pressed' oils. You can have fried foods on the ketogenic diet, but fry it in natural fats, like even lard and beef tallow, or duck fat, if you like to. Doesn't that sound pretty incredible?

Fish is also an excellent source of the right kinds of fats, so if you don't like fish, have fish oil capsules. If you do like seafood, you're in luck. This diet will keep you quite happy. Nuts like macadamia are also wonderful, and you can add peanut butter to your list of indulgences.

Here are a few ingredients you could stock up when you start the diet to get the right fats:

- Coconut oil
- Butter
- Avocados
- Peanut butter
- Coconut butter
- Ghee

- Macadamia nuts
- Duck fat
- Beef tallow
- Non-hydrogenated lard
- Cold-pressed vegetable oil

Proteins:

The original ketogenic diet has very little protein, but for weight loss, what you want is one that minimises your carbohydrate intake and has more fat and protein. You don't have to aim for a 4:1 ratio of fat to combined protein and carbs. A 1:1 ratio of protein to fat, cutting down carbs from grains as much as possible and having no added sugar at all, is a far more realistic aim. It's also an aim that will not leave you feeling unwell.

When it comes to protein, you have plenty of choice. You don't have to go out of your way to find lean cuts of protein, either. Feel like having chicken thighs instead of chicken breast? Go right ahead and pick it up. If you want to have bacon for breakfast, of course you can. Craving a sausage? You'll need to be sure there are no carbs as fillers in there, but if you can trust your butcher to give you real sausages, there is nothing to stop you from having it.

Eggs are also great, and the days of egg white omelettes are over. You can have eggs with yolk and know that you're still sticking to your diet. Most meat and fish will be fine on the ketogenic diet. Go ahead and get the fatty cuts if you feel like it. We'll go on to how you can get the portion sizes perfect, and remember that this diet will get you full faster than any other diet. Don't keep eating because it's tasty. Stop eating when you're full, and if you cook big batches and freeze, remember to divide it into appropriate portion sizes. If you cook each meal from scratch, weigh before you start and don't make any extra.

Here are a few things you can count on:

- Beef: steak, ground beef, anything you like.
- Hamburgers: make sure there are no fillers, of course.
- Chicken, any cut

- Duck
- Fish – salmon, trout, halibut, or most fishes you prefer
- Pork: chops, bacon, ham, belly, back – any kind you like
- Eggs, whole
- Shellfish
- Lamb: all cuts
- Quail
- Pheasant

Vegetables

You do need your greens. You need both the nutrients and the fibre. You will soon find out that life isn't like Man vs. Food. When I first embarked on this diet, I delighted at the thought of eating as much bacon as I wanted, but I soon realised that I didn't want as much bacon as I thought I did. The same followed for chops, sausages and burgers, my other favourite foods. I started looking forward to the vegetable part of the meals, so hit the farmer's market if you can every week, at least.

You can mix it up, but you need to be sure that you include lots of leafy green vegetables in your meals. Fruits, however, are more difficult. Most fruits have high levels of fructose, which is basically sugar, though naturally occurring, so care needs to be taken while choosing fruits.

Here are a few items you can't go wrong with:

- Lettuce
- Kale
- Bokchoy
- Cucumber
- Broccoli
- Asparagus
- Spinach
- Cauliflower
- Green beans
- Onions

- Mushrooms
- Bell pepper (but stick with green – coloured peppers are sweeter for the most obvious reason)
- Carrots
- Tomatoes

Remember that you can also have squash and snow peas, but not quite so frequently because they have slightly higher carb levels than the vegetables mentioned above. As a rule of thumb, if they're dark green and leafy, you can have them.

Nuts and seeds:

Nuts are good both as snacks and as garnish for your meals. Remember, though, that some of the nuts we take for granted are actually legumes – peanuts, for instance – and legumes are not part of the ketogenic diet. Here are the nuts you can safely have, though remember that moderation is key. It can be easy to forget you're chucking them in your mouth as you're engrossed in something else, but that shouldn't happen. Keep portion sizes in mind when you get your snack and you will have to stop when it's over. These are the nuts and seeds that are best for the diet:

- Macadamias
- Walnuts
- Almonds
- Chia seeds
- Flax seeds
- Hazelnuts
- Pecans

Cashew nuts and pistachios can be had in moderation since they're more carb-laden. One of the best parts about nuts is that almond flour can be used instead of plain flour for baking in some cases.

Dairy:

If you have resented every carton of low-fat milk and cheese you've bought so far, here's good news. You can get the full fat heavy cream, cheese and sour cream now. Go ahead and get full fat dairy products. Just the act of putting them in your shopping cart will make you feel light and happy. If you can, get organic everything. If you absolutely cannot, it cannot be helped. The ketogenic diet isn't only for those who can afford the organic lifestyle.

Drink:

This can be a problem. Most beverages have sugar in them. You're not supposed to have sugar. But you can live without sugar, right? Hopefully, you will be luckier than I was, since I quickly discovered that I had developed quite the addiction to sugar. But it was a challenge and I never back down from a challenge, so I made it work. If I could, so can you.

- Water. Drink more water. Then drink some more water. Drink a lot of water. Dehydration is a common problem with ketogenic diets, so drink lots and lots of water.
- Coffee – but drink more water to compensate for its diuretic effect.
- Tea – herbal or green, or even black. Cold green tea can be extremely refreshing.

Sweetening them up is a problem. You can go the artificial sweetener way, or you can use stevia or sucralose. I preferred the liquid forms since they were more likely to be pure and without additives.

No sugar. Absolutely no sugar.

Some people are of the opinion that an occasional glass of very dry wine is fine, and it probably is, but if you're going to stick with it for six weeks, do it well and go without the bottle, too.

Herbs and Spices

Don't buy any of the premixed spices or bottled dressings. Even if you buy spices separately and use the right measurements yourself, there will be carbohydrates in it. But you need flavour, and for flavour, you can use a light had with spices. Stock up on these:

- Sea salt instead of table salt
- Black pepper – get peppercorns and grind them yourself if you can
- Cayenne
- Chilli powder
- Coriander – seeds, to be dry roasted and powdered, and fresh
- Cumin – seeds, to be dry roasted and powdered when necessary
- Turmeric powder
- Sage
- Basil
- Rosemary
- Oregano
- Thyme

If you absolutely must get premixed packets, read the ingredients list properly and make sure that there is no added sugar in it. You will be surprised by how many have sugar.

You can use reasonable amounts of fresh garlic, but avoid powdered garlic and powdered onion. Allspice is also another thing to avoid. Yes, that will make it more difficult, but consider how much better your knowledge of flavours will get over the next six weeks! It will train your palate to recognise exactly what flavours combine beautifully, and that will be invaluable in every kind of cooking.

Things to remember:

No more tinned and canned stuff, and that includes even tomatoes. If you want to make a sauce, you will have to boil, blanch, peel and dice them yourself because canned tomatoes are loaded with sugar. Most things that come in jars have far too much sugar in them.

Fruits are a sticky point. You can have berries in very modest amounts, but they do have sugar. Avoid high-carb fruits as much as possible, and stick to berries. Remember you can have cream with it, though, so that should reduce the pain of not having the sweeter berries a bit.

Diet drinks are dangerous. They have artificial sweeteners, true, but they do cause you to have sugar cravings, and you end up trying to compensate for that. It's a bad idea altogether. Try to avoid them if you can, but if you must have soda, have diet soda.

Tricks to Beat Cravings

Even if you're supposed to feel full, cravings are another thing altogether. It doesn't matter how many duck breasts you have. There will be a part of you yelling 'where's the bread' inside you and trying to batter the door down. For me, more than bread, grains or refined starches, it was sugar. The morning caffeine kick just wasn't the same without the spoonful of sugar in it – pure glucose shot. It's the combination that gives me the jumpstart.

So whatever it might be, you do have your kryptonite. The good part is that you can control those cravings and fool them to a certain extent. The bad part is that some of it is psychological. You will have to pit your determination against the part of you that's urging you that one little piece of chocolate won't make a difference.

The first step is to identify what exactly your body is craving for. Yes, chocolate, but what within chocolate is making you feel like an addict going off crack who needs just one more fix?

If you're craving chocolate, what your body might be telling you is that it really wants some magnesium. Chocolate is an excellent way of getting magnesium if you're not on a diet. But if you're going ketogenic, then when you start dreaming of Mars Bars or Snickers, grab a handful of nuts and seeds instead. You will be surprised by how the intensity of your chocolate craving goes down when you have a few almonds.

Sugar is one of the biggest problems. If you've got used to having even a limited amount of sugar – and you have, the sheer quantity of hidden sugar we have is astounding once you start reading labels properly – you will be hit by sugar cravings. Don't fall into the trap of trying to sate it by having diet soda and other sugar-free sweet things. They intensify your craving because while your tongue is being satisfied, your body is not.

But let's break down the sugar craving. What your body is trying to get is a combination of minerals and nutrients that you can give it in other, healthy ways. Start with chromium, which is one of the biggest culprits as far as sugar cravings are concerned. Have a small wedge of cheese instead and you will feel a lot better. Broccoli can also help combat this craving, but cheese is a much nicer snack than broccoli when what you want is a doughnut.

Your body might also be demanding carbon, which you can give it if you have spinach. If it's sulphur, another possibility, then it's broccoli to the rescue again, though cauliflower florets can also do the trick. Phosphorous might be the problem. If so, beef, eggs and chicken are great options. Tryophan is yet another possibility, and cheese, liver and lamb can take care of that.

So when that sugar craving hits, you could just whip up a spinach and cheese omelette, and have a few broccoli florets to go with it. It's far healthier than a candy bar and much more satisfying, once you get your mind to stop obsessing over sweets and listen to what your body is trying to tell you.

Sometimes, when you sit down to a plate of really nice steak, you will feel yourself longing for a lasagne or a pizza. You're craving starch, but instead of giving in, have that steak and you will feel it getting less demanding. High protein meals like meat can alleviate that craving drastically.

Salty foods are another big draw. If you've got used to chips and dip, you will be hit by the craving. Dips are notorious for the amount of salt and sugar in it. But deal with it by giving your body fish, and another handful of seeds and nuts. You will begin to feel less driven by the craving.

Even if your body realises that it's got what it needed, your mind might still demand sugar and starch. One good way to take your mind off it is to drink lots of water. It will make you feel full, which in turn will control your cravings. Another little trick is to brush your teeth. Toothpaste can make all food taste absolutely dreadful. Once you have that aftertaste in your mouth, there's a good chance that your cravings will take second place.

A nice serving of shellfish grilled and tossed in butter, with sea salt and black pepper, is a lovely reward to give yourself for sticking it out and not giving in. It you're more of a meat person, you could make yourself a hamburger patty with ground beef and pork, and have that as a little reward. A lack of dips and sauces can make life a lot more boring, so read on, and once we get to recipes, we'll tackle that. They don't have to be fussy and they don't have to come out of bottles.

Meal Plan

If you're going on a ketogenic diet, it has to be a commitment. To make that kind of commitment, you have to be prepared. The first step, of course, is to inform yourself about the ketogenic diet. Then, once you have made a decision, you should get yourself checked out with a complete physical to be sure that you have no pre-existing condition that would affect you negatively if you go on this diet. It's also an excellent idea to consult a doctor and get his opinion as to how you will stand up to this diet.

Those are all common sense steps. If you're reading this, you're already well aware of all that, and if you've got this far, you know that you need a plan. Six weeks is a reasonable amount of time to plan for, so here's how you go about that.

First, you need to decide if you can trust your body to tell you when it's satisfied. With the ketogenic diet, one of the most common effects is that your body will feel nourished and full, so your appetite will naturally fall and you won't eat so much that you cannot maintain a calorie deficit. But there are exceptions to the rule, and what if you are one?

To be on the safe side, you could figure out what your macronutrient requirements are. Macros, as macronutrients are usually called because the full form is a real mouthful, that you need to think of are the three main groups: fats, proteins and carbohydrates. There are lots of calculators where you can input your details and find out how much of each you need. On average, for women, about 1600 calories a day is a good aim. Average split between macros is usually around 20 grams of carbohydrates, 136 grams of fat, and 74 grams of protein.

This could change according to your activity level and your metabolism, as well as your height and weight. Most of us work desk jobs and hop into the car or a bus for everything, so our lifestyles are fairly sedentary. If you are more active, please make sure that you calculate calories burnt accordingly and up your intake. If you are a tiny, pixie-like little thing, first, why are you trying to lose more weight; second, you will need to reduce your calorie intake unless your metabolism is extremely high.

If you need more calories, well, lucky you. Use lots of cream in your coffee, put an extra dollop of butter on your steak, have more bacon for breakfast – there are so many options when what you have to do is eat more! If you need fewer calories, well, join the club. Decreasing portion sizes so that both fat and protein intake go down in proportion is your best bet. Remember, there are calculators to use if you're unsure. You don't have to do the math yourself, and most of us are grateful for that!

But remember, counting calories on the ketogenic diet is something many people don't believe in at all. I didn't have to because I naturally ate less, so if you feel this is too little, keep your net carb intake low and have more of protein and fat. This meal plan will keep you both full and within that calorie intake range, but if you don't feel full, you can always add a snack or two. You can even use more of the main ingredient and eat more, and know that your decision is supported by a huge section of keto-followers. The calorie intake recommendation is mostly a nod to the common sense part that urges that you can't just abandon the logic of the calorie in-calorie out equation simply because the diet is ketogenic.

One thing you must remember is that this is a very strict diet as far as ingredients are concerned. You are free to play with the allowed ingredients, but you can't have just one cupcake because it looks so good. Unlike other diets, this depends on your body going into a different state, so it's not solely based on calories in versus calories out. A cheat meal can change the chemical balances you're hoping to induce in your body, and it can undo all the good work. Once you have reached your goal weight, of course, you can have more leeway, because you don't need to stay in a state of ketosis. But for the time you are on the diet, stick to it. Remember the craving defeating tricks, and we will give you recipes that will help you have cheats that aren't really cheats.

Six weeks can be a lot longer than you think, so be very sure that you mix your meals up, and be sure that you like what you eat. If you prefer red meat to fish, have fish oil capsules and red meat meals. Don't make yourself eat things you don't enjoy. The high-fat and high-protein food options are so vast that there is absolutely no reason why you should eat meals that you don't completely like.

Yet another thing before we start: you don't have to get exactly the number of macros you're supposed to every single day. You just need to average out right over three or four days. So you need to know how much of what is in every ingredient you use, but you don't need to get the calculator out for every meal and divide ingredients into unholy fractions.

You can always do the more basic recipes yourself. You can grill a steak, right? Well, that's perfectly fine, and you can just make sure that you have the right vegetables to go with it. If you're not sure, look it up. It's extremely easy to find the number of carbs in most vegetables. But remember that net carbs are total carbs minus the fibre weight.

Even if you do follow only the recommendations here, your macros will not be exactly what is recommended. But your net carbs will be lower than the recommended maximum, so you will definitely be in ketosis, and your calorie consumption might be just a bit lower than the recommended maximum.

Now, it's up to you to use your common sense a lot of the time. If you feel like just frying up some bacon and having a boiled egg in the morning, go for it. It's perfectly fine. Keep the bacon grease and fry a steak for dinner, and take a bagged salad for lunch with one of the dressings. If you feel full halfway through a meal even if you haven't had the entire serving size, pack it up and keep it in the fridge. Most of these recipes will last for a few days if you keep them packed properly.

Since steaks, fried eggs, bacon, slices of ham, boiled eggs, grilled fish and so on are ubiquitous, such recipes have not been included in the book. If you're old enough to decide to go on the ketogenic diet, you must be self aware enough to know what flavour combinations you like on basic foods like grilled meat and fish, or stir-fried or steamed shellfish. When you already have a favourite way of making those basic dishes, it would be an insult to tell you how to make it my way.

But the exception is pork chops, since the low-fat way of cooking has made most of us too reluctant to use butter with pork chops. Use butter and coconut oil with anything you feel like. Fish, for instance, is wonderful made in coconut oil. You know that coconuts palms are part of coastal landscape – it's one of nature's ways of telling us to use the oil to make the fish you get from the sea.

If you make the lamb stew or something similarly involved one day, have leftovers for breakfast. There's no rule that says that you can't have a microwave egg cup for dinner. As long as you count your carbs, mixing and matching is up to you. For most of these recipes, even if you combine the heaviest ones for one day, you'll find it difficult to have more than 22 grams of carbs a day. You will also find it very difficult to move after you're done eating because those meals are very heavy.

To keep from plateauing, there is a straightforward thing you can do: fast. Week 1 will see you dropping weight fairly easily, though you may feel pretty horrible. Grit your teeth and power through it. Week 2 will be easier, but you will stop losing weight quite so steadily.

So get tough on Weeks 3 and 4: have a fat-heavy shake for breakfast, with or without caffeine, according to your choice; skip lunch – yes, skip lunch, that's why it's called fasting – and have a heavier than usual dinner. Increase the portion size if you don't feel full after what you're used to having.

Week 5, go back to three meals a day, and use your creativity. Now you know how to work with these ingredients. You know how to make ketogenic meals. So experiment, and have fun.

Week 6, mix it up by fasting again. But keep things interesting by adding new things to your meals, like, for instance, zucchini noodles. Make desserts. I promise you, you will find that your tastebuds have undergone a radical change, and keto desserts will taste incredible.

After that, you will be on your own, but the good part about not giving you a strictly regimented meal plan for six weeks is that you will know, by then, how to get creative. You will have a stable of reliable recipes, but you will also have learnt to mix it up to choose your palate. Remember, this is your life. There is no point going on a diet for six weeks if it makes you miserable.

Two days' worth of meal plan demos are given for each week, and that should give you the added entertainment of flipping through the recipes and deciding on one that looks particularly appealing to you. Follow the same model to plan your meals for the rest of the day, count your carbs, and listen to your body. Once you're comfortable enough, tweak the recipes to your tastes. Find more and experiment. As long as you count carbs and make sure that your protein intake isn't far outweighing your fat intake – remember, fatty cuts of meat will solve a lot of that problem – you can get really inspired. Now that rice, pasta and bread are all out of the question, just imagine how much more interesting it can be to play with ingredients that are more than just fillers!

So now to our first step: Get the ingredients.

If you need desserts, there are a few ingredients you need to get now. If you can get it at your local supermarket, that's great. If you can't, however, you will need to order them. At least by week two, you should be able to cook with all ingredients, so get almond flour, liquid stevia, coconut oil and flour, milled flaxseed meal and an additional sweetener, erythritol. This could get very boring without those ingredients, so get ordering now.

Before you go shopping, check your staples. Then make a list, using this as reference:

- Meat:
    - Bacon (save the fat when you cook it, though)
    - Pork rinds and chops
    - Chicken thighs
    - Beef: ground, steaks, stew cut
    - Sausages, especially chorizo
    - Lamb: stew cut
- Fish:
    - Canned fish without additives
    - Shrimp, shelled
- Fats:
    - Heavy cream
    - Half and half
    - Salted and unsalted butter (grassfed would be better)
    - Oliver oil, preferably extra virgin
    - Coconut oil
    - Lard
    - Cheese: cheddar, cream, Parmesan, Mozzarella
- Vegetables
    - Spinach – lots, lots, lots and more spinach
    - Green pepper
    - Onions – you can get quite a bit since onions keep fairly well
    - Broccoli
    - Sugar snap peas
    - Cauliflower
    - Green beans

- - Parsley
  - Cucumber
  - Coriander, fresh
  - Tomato
  - Green chilli
  - Button mushrooms
  - Lemons
  - Spring onion
- Spices
  - Black pepper
  - Sea salt
  - Cayenne pepper
  - Chilli powder
  - Turmeric powder
  - Coriander, seeds and powder
  - Cumin, seeds and powder
  - Ginger
  - Garlic
  - Oregano
  - Thyme
  - Basil
  - Rosemary
  - Sage
  - Bay leaf
  - Cardamom
  - Cloves
  - Cinnamon
  - Xanthan gum
- Extras:
  - Coconut milk
  - Full fat yoghurt
  - Beef broth
  - Chicken stock

- o   Red wine, dry
- o   White wine, dry
- o   Dijon mustard (check the label carefully)
- o   Worcestershire sauce
- o   Fish sauce (go gluten-free)
- o   Vinegar
- o   Soy sauce
- o   Almonds
- o   Sesame seeds
- o   Pecans
- o   Pumpkin seeds

Remember that most of these spices will last you a while, so this will be the first big shopping trip. Don't get intimidated. There are a lot of spices simply because it's better to buy them individually than to get the ubiquitous 'curry powder' packets that will have additives and more flavouring agents. You want to know what's going into your body, remember. It will all be worth it, in the long run.

Calorie and macro counts are given with the recipes, so make sure you adjust your portions accordingly for each meal.

When you have six weeks to get through, there are a few adjustments to be made. For instance, once you have gone into ketosis in the first couple of weeks, you could plateau. One of the best ways to get out of that is to load up on fats during breakfast, and then fast. Ketosis, science suggests, is how the body deals with starvation. So while we won't starve, missing one meal to make your body believe that you're deprived of food might be beneficial to you. If it doesn't work for you, go back to the breakfast recipes. But be sure you adjust the carbs allowed for dinner, especially dessert – yes, you got that right, dessert – if you do that.

Week 1
This will be the toughest week, but I promise you, it will get better. Don't try anything too fancy in the kitchen this week. The stress of trying to figure out a whole new way of cooking while dealing with the expected side effects of ketosis can be overwhelming. So keep it simple and drink as much water as you possibly can. Forget the two litres a day.

Double that if you can. You will also be losing electrolytes, so you can put a pinch of salt in your water, as well. You will get headaches, feel sick and exhausted, both physically and mentally. Think of the fabulous body you will have soon and hold on.

Make sure you don't go to places without a bathroom, because you will have to pee a lot. Try not to make important appointments because brain fogginess is to be expected. Don't start the ketogenic diet when there's an important deal to be made at work or your kids have got exams coming up. All this will combine to make you quite irritable, so warn your partner that they will have to put up with a few bouts of short-tempered nastiness. I buried myself in books, music and movies as much as I could, and took my temper out on inanimate objects. Find your outlets. It's important.

Take as much pleasure as you can in your shopping trip, because all those things you wouldn't get when you were on low-fat diets are good for you now. Get the butter, the bacon, the full fat cream cheese. Yes, I said the 'full fat cream cheese'. You're free to have it.

Day 1:

Breakfast: Cheese and mushroom scrambled eggs with bacon

Lunch: Salad (with lots of spinach and a grilled chicken breast)

> Remember that you can mix up your salad by changing the ingredients and seasoning. Choose one from the many dressings you will learn to make, quickly and easily. If you didn't have time or ran out, remember that olive oil and lemon juice with some salt and pepper is a simple and effective dressing, too.

Dinner: Lamb stew

> Don't forget that the recipe isn't for one person! You can freeze this in portions and it will fine. No, it's not the same without potatoes, but such are the sacrifices that must be made. You won't miss then when you're eating, though.

Day 2

Breakfast: Microwave Egg Cups

Yes, microwave can be gourmet, and anybody who disagrees can go take a hike. If it tastes good to you, what's the big deal?

Lunch: Salad with lots of greens and chorizo

The sour cream dressing goes wonderfully well with this, though the plain vinaigrette works as well.

Dinner: Lamb stew / Grilled steak with French beans and asparagus

If you don't feel like having leftovers, grilling a steak is really easy to do. Fry the beans and asparagus in the same skillet for added flavour.

Week 2

By now you must have got a bit used to being in ketosis, and you should be seeing how the pounds have started melt of you. Kilograms, too, if you follow the metric system. Your brain fog should have lifted, and you should be feeling a lot more up to something that takes a bit of effort. So reward yourself with some waffles. Yes, we did say waffles. And you can use the leftover waffles as sandwich bread tomorrow for lunch. Sandwiches again! You will also have noticed by now that there is more sweetness in food that doesn't have conventionally sweet ingredients than you'd imagined. It hit me very hard, and after the diet, I never went back to the spoonful of sugar in my coffee again.

Day 8

Breakfast: Coconut Flour Waffles

> Remember, if you make extra, you will have leftovers for breakfast the next day, too. Stored in an airtight container, they will keep easily for a few days. Add a dollop of butter if you're feeling decadent. You made it a week, you deserve it.

Lunch: Grilled chicken salad with lettuce, a cucumber, carrot and broccoli.

> Use the vinaigrette for dressing because breakfast was pretty heavy.

Dinner: Keto Chili

> Don't eat all of it at one sitting if you can stop yourself. Freeze it. You'll be glad when you're too tired to make anything for dinner, and you know that day is inevitable every week.

Day 9

Breakfast: Cheese and mushroom scrambled eggs

> Back to basics, and it's much faster than waffles. Besides, leftover waffles for lunch!

Lunch: Waffles and chorizo sandwich with lettuce and cucumber

Sandwich lunch again – did you think you'd be so excited for a sandwich lunch? A few carrot sticks will make sure you get your nutrients, too.

Dinner: Spiced Baked Chicken Thighs

It looks fancy but it's extremely easy. It's also very filling and extremely tasty, so it ticks all the boxes.

Week 3

Week 2 was easy, wasn't it? You were coasting along, having fun making pancakes and waffles, trying new recipes and deciding that this ketogenic thing is a breeze, after all. Now we get to the first real road block. You will have ketogenic high-fat shakes for breakfast, fast through lunch, and have a heavy dinner. The good part is that desserts may be had as long as you are within your carb limits.

Now this might sound intimidating, but remember how intimidating that first week of going on the ketogenic diet was? But now you're an old hand at it. So stiffen those sinews and stick it out, because there are desserts at the end of it.

Day 15

Breakfast: Keto Caffeine Blast

> The caffeine will help you survive. Listen to experience, and have the caffeine the first day.

Lunch: Water. Water is good. Had water already? That's great, have more water.

Dinner: Stuffed pork chops

> This is an extremely filling and extremely satisfying dinner, and you will be happy for it.

Dessert: Peanut butter cup

> They're not strictly the best thing for the moment, but you deserve the treat. Freeze the remaining before you gobble them up.

Day 16

Breakfast: Keto Shake

> Pick a shake that you think will keep you as satisfied as possible. If the caffeine worked, stick with it.

Lunch: Remember water? Meet water again. You're best buddies now.

Dinner: Hot and sour pork with pepper

This will make you forget that you didn't have lunch, it's that good. Increase portion size if you find it's not filling enough. Be lulled into the hot and sour pork stupor.

Week 4

By now, the fasting should be a piece of cake to you. If you feel like having a proper breakfast, go right ahead and whip something up, but remember to add an extra dollop of butter to all of it. You need more fat. Did you ever think you would hear that on a diet? You need more fat!

Day 22

Breakfast: Keto Caffeine Blast

> This is the lowest carb smoothie in the recipes. If you manage to vary and change another into something similar, go for it.

Lunch: Zilch.

Dinner: Crockpot pork

> Have a small stir-fried vegetable salad or a fresh salad to go with this, because you need your vitamins.

Day 23

Breakfast: Avocado-coconut smoothie

> Remember, you can always add different flavours to your smoothies. It's one of the easiest things to play with.

Lunch: We did talk about how important water is, right?

Dinner: Chicken and chorizo stew

> Again, a fresh salad with lots of greens would be excellent to go with this. Go on and have dessert, too. The spiced mug cakes are easy and yummy.

Week 5

You're back on the breakfast wagon now, so celebrate with pancakes. After all, you deserve it, don't you? It's been an entire month and you've managed to stick with the ketogenic diet. Of course, by now, you're also probably coming to the conclusion that it really was not such a big deal. You should be seeing the weight shed, and now you can consider adding an exercise regimen to tone up, as well. You're losing fat, which is great. Now maybe it's time to consider toning up the muscles. Remember to adjust your food intake according to your activity level, again.

Day 29

Breakfast: Almond flour pancakes

> This really is a winner, especially with some extra butter on top.

Lunch: Greens salad with avocado and sour cream dressing.

> Just combine the two and adjust seasonings. You should be an old hand at this by now!

Dinner: Stuffed peppers

> If there's a part of you that misses rice even now, it won't after the stuffed peppers. They're a real miracle.

Day 30

Breakfast: Ham and cheese scrambled eggs

> Filling, easy and delicious.

Lunch: Leftover crockpot

> From the week before – you still have some left, right? Making bigger batches means a lot less work!

Dinner: Stuffed chicken breast

> Far easier than it looks, and it works for company, too, if you make two.

Week 6

This is your last week on the ketogenic diet. Even if you plan to keep up with the low-carbohydrate diet, you will want to start adjusting your calorie intake and your macro nutrient distribution to whatever you want it to be as you go on. If you decide to stick with it, going on from week five, with a few desserts, will work just great. If you decide to add more carbs you will need to start cutting down on your fat intake slowly and have more protein and vegetable carbs. You could try having fruits, as well. Remember, keeping your body in ketosis forever is not a very realistic ideal, but cutting down on your carbohydrates intake is beneficial. Find a middle ground that works for you.

Day 36

Breakfast: Cheese and mushroom scrambled eggs

> This works on every diet. If there's a diet that doesn't allow this breakfast, the diet shouldn't be allowed to exist.

Lunch: Salad with chorizo and grilled chicken breast, with yoghurt dressing

> By now, you have got so used to your diet that having carbs for lunch will make you feel heavy. Even if you do decide to add carbs to your diet, do it for breakfast, not lunch.

Dinner: Steamed shellfish

> Of course, you have to get fresh shellfish, but if you can, it's an excellent meal with loads of butter!

Day 37

Breakfast: Coconut flour waffles

> You must be a dab hand at whipping them up by now, so it will barely take any time.

Lunch: Waffle sandwich with bacon and lettuce

> See, you don't need carbs for lunch after all!

Dinner: Traditional pork chops

Again an easy meal to make, so it's a no-fuss day.

By the time you're done with Week 6, you will have a few decisions to make. Try on those clothes that you couldn't fit into earlier, admire yourself, revel in how fit you feel, and remember, it's your choice how you go on. To keep this weight off, stay on a low-carb diet, build a reasonable activity level and stay away from sugar and starches. Give yourself room for a few cheats here and there, but keep them far and few between.

So now you're on your own, but you can always come back for quick reference. And keep the recipes – they're winners.

Recipes

Breakfast recipes:

Cheesy scrambled eggs

Net Carb Count: 1.1 grams

Ingredients:

Whole eggs	2
Butter	1 Tbsp
Cheddar cheese	1 ounce
Salt and pepper	to taste
Spring onion shoots	to garnish

Method:

- Heat skillet on your stove and slide the butter into it. Let it melt.
- Break the two eggs into a bowl, add salt and pepper to taste, then whip it. Grate the cheddar cheese into it and whip it again.
- Lower the heat and pour the egg mixture into the skillet. Stirring occasionally to keep it fluffy, let the eggs cook slowly. Chop the shoots of the spring onions.
- Once they are cooked how you like it, transfer to your plate and garnish with chopped spring onion shoots.

Cheese and mushroom scrambled eggs

Net Carb Count: 2.1 grams

Ingredients

Whole eggs	2
Cheddar cheese	1 ounce
Butter	2 Tbsp
Button mushrooms, sliced	½ cup
Salt and pepper	to taste

Method:

- Heat the skillet and let the butter melt. Add the mushrooms and let them fry till they begin to show a good golden colour

- Meanwhile, whip the eggs with grated cheese, salt and pepper.

- Lower the heat on the skillet and add the whipped eggs. On low heat, let it cook slowly, stirring just enough to keep it scrambled.

Ham and cheese scrambled eggs

Net Carb Count: 1.1 grams

Ingredients:

Whole eggs	2
Ham	1 slice
Cheddar cheese	1 ounce
Butter	1 Tbsp
Salt and pepper	to taste

Method:

- Heat the skillet and let the butter melt. Shred the ham roughly and add it to the butter.

- Meanwhile, whip the eggs with grated cheese, salt and pepper.

- Lower the heat on the skillet and add the whipped eggs. On low heat, let it cook slowly, stirring just enough to keep it scrambled.

Almond flour pancakes (makes 4 servings)

Net Carb Count (per serving) 4.4 grams

Ingredients

Almond flour	1.5 cups
Eggs, whole	3
Water	¾ cup
Heavy cream	¼ cup
Stevia	to taste

Method

- Whip all the ingredients for the batter together. You can whip by hand if you feel up to it. Make sure it's smooth and easy to pour. Add more water if you need to thin it out.

- Taste the batter and add stevia to your preference. Be careful to add by the drop. The pancakes turn out fine without an additional sweetener, too, but you're supposed to enjoy your meal. Meanwhile, heat the griddle.

- Make one test pancake to judge sweetness as well as texture. Adjust batter if required, then make the rest.

- Wrap in clingfilm and refrigerate to keep for a few days.

Coconut Flour Waffles (makes 8)

Net Carb Count per serving (2 waffles): 2.275 grams

Ingredients:

Coconut flour	one ounce
Heavy cream	2 Tbsp
Stevia extract	to taste
Eggs, whole	6
Sea salt	a pinch
Water	as necessary

Method

- Preheat the waffle iron. High heat does no harm.

- Mix all the ingredients together until it's smooth and the consistency is right. Be careful with the stevia extract, as usual.

- Pour the batter onto the waffle iron and smooth it over with a spatula or a butter knife. Close the iron and let it cook for three to four minutes. When it's golden brown, it's done.

- Have it with a pat of butter if you feel like something extra!

Cheesy egg muffins (serves four)

Net Carb Count: 2.6 grams

Ingredients

Eggs, whole	8
Half and half	½ cup
Bacon (cooked and chopped)	4 ounce
Cheddar cheese	½ cup
Butter	1 Tbsp
Parsley	a small handful
Salt and pepper	to taste

Method

- Preheat the oven to 375 degrees Fahrenheit. Grease a muffin tray well with butter.

- In a bowl, crack the eggs and add the half and half, whipping together till it looks almost scrambled. Then fold in the cooked and chopped bacon, whatever spices you feel like adding, and cheese.

- Pour the batter into eight muffin cups in the tray. If there are empty cups, fill them with water. Each cup should be about three-quarters full.

- Bake for about 15 minutes, waiting a few more minutes if they're not golden around the edges.

- Once they're out of the oven, let them cool for a minute. Eat one or two immediately and wrap the rest in clingfilm and freeze.

Microwave Egg Cup

Net carb count: 3 grams

Ingredients

Eggs, whole	2
Ham	1 slice
Shallots	1 Tbsp
Cheddar cheese	1 ounce
Half and half	½ Tbsp
Salt and pepper	to taste

Method:

- Grease one microwave-safe coffee mug with butter.

- Crack the eggs and whip them with salt and pepper to taste. Add the half and half, whip again without overdoing it.

- Pour it into the mug and put it in the microwave, medium setting, for a minute.

- Take it out, add shredded ham, shallots and cheese (grated), stir, pop it back in the microwave for about 45 seconds.

Lunch & Dinner Recipes

Lamb Stew (serves four)

Net Carb Count per serving: 5.2 grams

Ingredients

Lamb, preferably shoulder	1 pound
Onion	¼ medium, chopped
Garlic	2 cloves, minced
Cinnamon	2 inches
Cloves	4
Cardamom	4
Coconut milk	250 ml
Salt and pepper	to taste
Green beans	½ pound
Coconut oil	2 Tbsp

Method

- In a skillet, heat the coconut oil. Add the whole spices, and then the minced garlic. Let the garlic brown well. Now add the chopped onion and let it brown.

- Into the skillet, add the lamb and let it brown well. Lower the heat.

- Add half the coconut milk and enough water to just cover the meat. Cover and let it simmer for about half an hour or 45 minutes, till the lamb is deliciously tender.

- Add the green beans and wait a couple of minutes till they're cooked but still have a slight bite to them.

- Add salt and pepper to taste, then, still on low heat, add the remainder of the coconut milk and let it just come to a simmer. Turn it off and remove from heat.

Baked and Spiced Chicken Thighs

Net Carb Count: 1.4 grams

Ingredients

Chicken thighs	2
Garlic	1 clove, minced
Ginger	¼ inch, minced
Chilli powder	1/8 tsp
Cayenne pepper	1/8 tsp
Coriander powder	1/8 tsp
Cumin	1/8 tsp
Salt and pepper	to taste
Olive oil	1 Tbsp + 1 tsp
Lemon	juice of one wedge

Method

- Rub all the ingredients except 1 tsp of olive oil on the chicken thighs. Let it marinate, covered, in the fridge for an hour.

- Preheat the oven to 425 degrees Fahrenheit.

- Cover a baking pan with foil and pour a teaspoon of olive oil to coat.

- Place the chicken thighs on the tray and bake for about 25 minutes. Then flip the chicken thighs and bake till done, another 15-20 minutes.

Hot and Sour Pork with Peppers (makes four servings)

Net Carb Count per serving : 2 grams

Ingredients

Pork shoulder	½ pound, julienned
Green pepper	1, julienned
Green/Red chilli	1 or 2
Garlic	4 cloves, minced
Soy sauce	3 Tbsp
White vinegar	¼ cup
Chicken stock	1 cup
Oil (coconut or olive or sesame)	2 Tbsp
Pepper	to taste

Method

- In a wok, heat the oil. Add minced garlic and finely sliced chilli – one if using green, two if using red.
- Add the pork and on high heat, flash fry for two minutes.
- Add soy sauce, chicken broth and vinegar, let it simmer till the pork is cooked.
- Turn up the heat and add the julienned pepper. Let the liquid evaporate till you get your preferred consistency.
- Taste, season with pepper if you want it to be spicier.

You can modify this recipe by adding different kinds of mushrooms instead of pepper. You can also use bamboo shoot and more chicken stock, stirring in whipped egg once it's done, for a soupier meal. Use a fattier cut of pork if you feel like it, too, but keep an eye on the cholesterol!

Chorizo and Beef Meatballs (Makes three generous servings)

Net Carb Count per serving: 3.3 grams

Ingredients

Ground beef	1 pound
Chorizo sausages	1 pound
Crushed pork rinds	½ cup
Egg	2
Cumin	½ tsp
Salt	to taste
Pepper	to taste
Parmesan cheese	1 cup
Tomatoes, sliced	1 cup

Method

- Chop up and crumble the chorizo sausages to make it easy to mix with the rest of the ingredients.

- Preheat the oven to 350 degrees Fahrenheit.

- Mix all ingredients except cheese and tomatoes in a bowl. Be careful not to overmix.

- Grease an oven tray.

- Make a dozen big balls out of the mix, arrange on the tray.

- Bake for about 20 minutes, then take out of the oven and top each with a slice of tomato and a bit of cheese. Pop back in the oven till meatballs are done.

Stuffed Chicken Breast

Net Carb Count: 2.9 grams

Ingredients

Chicken breast	1, medium
Spinach	1 cup, chopped
Salt and pepper	to taste
Mozzarella cheese	¼ cup
Lemon	juice of ½
Oregano	½ tsp

Method

- Pound the chicken breast, but not too hard. You want it to get a bit flatter so it's easier to stuff, but not so flat that you have to roll it. Pat the chicken completely dry. Rub it with salt, pepper and half the oregano.
- In a saucepan or skillet, whichever is handy, wilt the spinach so that most of the moisture runs free. Squeeze it through a kitchen towel in a sieve. If you're feeling very healthy, you could just drink it.
- Preheat the oven to 350 degrees Fahrenheit.
- Mix the wilted spinach, cooled, with the grated mozzarella cheese, the remaining oregano, and salt and pepper to taste. Cut a slit down the side of the chicken breast and stuff it with the mixture.
- Place it in a greased or foil-covered oven tray and squeeze the lemon over it. Coat it with olive oil and cook till juices run clear.

You can add walnuts to the stuffing for a different flavour and texture. You could also drop a dollop of butter on the chicken breast for the last couple of minutes in the oven for extra yumminess. There might be leftover filling, but it works great as a side dish to go with the stuffed chicken breast.

Stuffed Chicken Thigh

Net Carb Count: 1 gram

Ingredients

Chicken thighs, boneless	2
Chorizo sausage, chopped	¼ cup
Mushroom, chopped	¼ cup
Cheddar cheese	¼ cup
Salt and pepper	to taste
Olive oil	3 Tbsp

Method

- Preheat the oven to 350 degrees Fahrenheit.

- Pat the chicken thighs dry very well.

- In a skillet, pour a tablespoon of olive oil and brown the mushrooms thoroughly.

- In a bowl, combine the sausage, mushroom, cheddar cheese, salt and pepper.

- Scoop as much of the stuffing as the chicken thigh can hold and still be folded over onto the thigh. Fold over and pin with toothpicks. Use the remaining stuffing as a side.

- Rub salt, pepper and olive oil on the chicken thighs.

- Place in an oven tray with the rest of the olive oil and bake for about 20 minutes, covered in foil. Remove foil and bake till juice runs clear and chicken is browned.

Note: You can use one minced clove of garlic, added to the skillet before mushrooms and browned, if you like the flavour of garlic. It's not necessary for the dish to taste great, but it can add a great hit.

Beef and wine stew (makes four comfortable servings)

Net Carb Count (per serving) : 8 grams

Ingredients

Beef (your choice of cut for stew)	2 pounds
Onion, finely chopped	1 medium
Dry red wine	10 ounces
Bay leaf	2
Bacon	100 gm
Carrots	2 large
Thyme	½ tsp
Garlic, minced	3 cloves
Salt and pepper	to taste
Butter, unsalted	1 Tbsp
Parsley, fresh	a handful

Method

- Preheat the oven to 350 degrees Fahrenheit and find a cast iron casserole that can go in the oven. This is the most time-consuming part of the recipe, I promise.

- In the cast iron casserole, melt the butter and brown the beef, cut into cubes, well. Add the onion and garlic, stirring enough so nothing gets burnt, for about five minutes. Now add the thyme, bay leaves and wine. Season with salt and pepper, let it come to a boil and make sure you scrape all the nice, caramelised brown bits down from the sides.

- Cover and put it in the oven for about an hour and a half.

- In a saucepan with a bit of olive oil, add the bacon and let it cook. Add the carrots, sliced, to that, and add some pepper, too. Turn the heat down low and let it cook, covered, till the carrots are soft.

- Add the bacon and carrots to the stew once you take it out of the oven, stir, garnish with parsley. Try not to eat it all.

Pork Chops Grilled with Soy Sauce and Red Chilli

Net Carb Count: .5 grams

Ingredients

Pork chops	2
Garlic, minced	2 cloves
Soy sauce	1 Tbsp
Vinegar, white	1 Tbsp
Red chilli, minced	1

Method

- Rub the pork chops thoroughly with all the ingredients.

- Grill them on the stove till they're done. It will depend on the thickness of the chops, but 11 minutes is usually adequate.

Note: Use a dry white wine to deglaze the pan if you'd like a sauce to go with it.

Stuffed Pork Chops

Net Carb Count: 3 grams

Ingredients

Pork chops, 2 inches thick	2
Bacon slices	3
Cheddar cheese	¼ cup
Cream cheese	¼ cup
Spring onion shoots	½ cup
Garlic, minced	1 clove

Method

- Go to the butcher and ask for your pork chops to be sliced thick. Don't worry. Butchers don't use their giant knives and other weapons of mass destruction on people.

- Preheat the oven to 350 degrees Fahrenheit.

- Cook the bacon in a skillet, with half the garlic. Reserve the bacon grease to brown the chops and chop up the bacon into fairly small pieces.

- In a bowl, combine chopped spring onion shoots, bacon and both cheeses.

- Stand the chops up, with the fatty sides down, and slice them. Stuff everything in the bowl into them. Now rub them well with the remaining garlic and salt and pepper.

- Brown the chops in the bacon grease and transfer to an oven-proof dish if your skillet is not oven proof. Bake for about 45 minutes, or use a meat thermometer. Let it rest for three minutes before digging in or you will lose all the juices.

Note: Net carb count is for both chops. Yes, serving size is one. But these are ridiculously good. I felt perfectly full at half a chop, and ended up eating two. It was a horribly uncomfortably full few hours but the next time I made it, I did it again. Divide by two if you eat only one, you embodiment of astonishing will power, you.

Traditional Pork Chops

Total carb count: with accompaniments, 7 grams; without, negligible

Ingredients

Pork chops	2
Rosemary	½ tsp
Salt and pepper	to taste
Butter	1 Tbsp

Method

- Rub the rosemary, salt and pepper well into the pork chops.
- In a skillet, melt the butter. Turn it on medium-high heat and place the chops in the skillet. Once it's browned, flip the chops and lower the heat for about 12 minutes or until completely cooked.

Note: Serve this with blanched asparagus and green beans, and carrots fried in the same pan, if you'd like accompaniments.

Stuffed Peppers

Net Carb Count: 10 grams

Ingredients

Green pepper	2
Butter	1 Tbsp
Onion, chopped	1/8 medium
Garlic, minced	1 clove
Shaved steak	½ pound
Salt and pepper	to taste
Cheddar cheese	¼ cup

Method

- Preheat the oven to 400 degrees Fahrenheit.
- Cut the tops of the peppers off. Deseed them and chop up what you have from the top part. Place the cup parts of the peppers on a foil covered, greased tray in the oven until just soft.
- In a skillet, melt the butter and add the garlic, chopped green pepper and onion. Stir till soft, then add the seasoning and shaved steak. Use your spatula to make sure it's in small pieces and let it cook all the way through.
- Distribute the cheddar cheese between the two pepper cups. Top with the stuffing and put them back in the oven for about three to five minutes.

Note: If you don't eat the pepper cup, you will avoid about 4 grams of carbs per pepper. If you eat one whole and only the stuffing of the other, this meal will only be 6 grams of carbs.

Veggie Night

Net Carb Count: 7.8 grams

Ingredients

Butter	3 Tbsp
Broccoli	115 grams
Green pepper	90 grams
Spinach	150 grams
Pumpkin seeds	2 Tbsp
Garlic, minced	3 cloves
Cumin	one pinch
Cayenne pepper	one pinch
Salt and pepper	to taste
Mushrooms (mix them up)	240 grams

Method

- Let the butter melt in the skillet, then add the minced garlic. Add the mushrooms, let it sauté; then add cumin.
- Now add the peppers, broccoli, sugar snap peas and the rest of the spices and seasoning.
- After a few seconds, add the pumpkin seeds. Now put the spinach on top and cover for a minute or two so that it's wilted well.
- Stir well and serve.

Chicken and Chorizo: One Pot Stew (8 very comfortable servings)

Net Carb Count: 5 grams

Ingredients

Chicken thighs	4 pounds
Chorizo	1 pound
Tomatoes	1 pound
Chicken stock	3 cups
Garlic, minced	12 cloves
Ginger, minced	2 inches
Heavy cream	1 cup
Salt and pepper	to taste
Worcestershire sauce	1 Tbsp
Red chilli	2
Sour cream and Parmesan	to garnish

Method:

- Boil, blanch, peel, deseed and chop the tomatoes.
- In a skillet, use some butter to brown the chorizo. Follow up by browning the chicken thighs.
- In the crock pot, start layering: chicken goes first, then the chorizo, then the spices and sauces.
- Cook on high for about three hours. By then, the chicken should be perfect to fall apart. Pull them into small strips and turn it down to low for another half an hour.
- Garnish and serve.

Keto Chili (makes four servings)

Net Carb Count (per serving): 5.4 grams

Ingredients

Stew meat	1 pound
Ground meat	1 pound
Green pepper	1
Tomato	2
Garlic, minced	2 cloves
Soy sauce	2 Tbsp
Olive oil	2 Tbsp
Chili powder	2 Tbsp + 1 tsp, but more if you really like spice
Cumin	2 tsp
Paprika	1 Tbsp
Fish Sauce	2 tsp
Oregano	1 tsp
Cayenne pepper	1 tsp
Worcestershire sauce	1 tsp

Method:

- Chop all the veggies fairly finely.

- Boil, blanch, skin and deseed tomatoes, then blitz them into a paste.

- Brown first the cubes of meat, then the ground beef, and put in a slow cooker.

- In the same pan, sauté all the vegetables till the onions are nice and translucent.

- Add everything to the slow cooker, including the sauces and spices, then turn it to high and let it cook for at least two hours. Then lower the heat and simmer for about half an hour.

Note: You can change the quantities of hot seasoning however you like!

Keto Crockpot Pork (Makes four comfortable servings)

Net Carb Count (per serving): 2.5 grams

Ingredients

Pork butt	2 pounds
Butter	½ Tbsp
Onion, thinly sliced	¼
Cumin	½ Tbsp
Thyme	1 Tbsp
Chilli powder	1 Tbsp
Garlic, minced	4 cloves
Chicken stock	¼ cup
Salt and pepper	to taste

Method

- Coat the crockpot with butter, then layer the onion at the bottom. Sprinkle the garlic on top of that.

- Cutting the very fatty part off the pork, score the meat. Rub the spices into it very well. Place it in the crockpot.

- Add the chicken stock, and whatever spices are left, and cook on high heat for about two hours.

Dressings and Dips

First of all, learn how to make a quick tahini at home. You can store it in the fridge in an airtight container for up to a couple of weeks. There are very few dressings that can't be given a good punch with a teaspoon of tahini. Even plain sour cream, combined with some tahini and cayenne pepper, can be a wonderful salad dressing. It's one of those things where a little goes a long way, though, so don't overdo it.

Tahini

Total Net Carb Count (for all of it): 16 grams

Ingredients

White sesame seeds   1 cup

Olive oil   4 Tbsp

Salt   a tiny pinch, optional.

Method

- In a skillet, lightly toast the sesame seeds. Be careful not to burn them – they burn quite easily. If you burn them, there's no saving them.

- Transfer the toasted sesame seeds onto a flat tray and let them cool completely.

- Put the sesame seeds in a food processer and let it be ground to a crumbly texture, for about 45 seconds to a minute.

- Now add the olive oil and continue to blend. It could take up to four or five minutes, and you will need to scrape the sides off regularly.

- Add salt if you wish and let it blend for a few more seconds.

- Store in an airtight container.

Cool Yoghurt Dressing (four generous servings)

Carb Count (per serving): 2 grams

Ingredients

Full fat yoghurt	150 gm
Olive oil	2 Tbsp
Tahini	1 Tbsp
Cayenne pepper	½ tsp
Salt	one pinch
Garlic	1 clove

Method

- Toast the garlic and mince it very finely.

- Add all the ingredients together and whip till uniformly mixed. Add more olive oil to change the consistency to suit you.

Sour Cream Dip

Net Carb Count: 3.7 grams

Ingredient

Sour Cream	½ cup
Heavy cream	¼ cup
Parsley, chopped	3 Tbsp
Dill, chopped	1 tsp
Garlic, minced	1 clove, roasted
Salt and pepper	to taste

Method:

Whip all the ingredients together. If you'd like it to keep longer than a couple of days, use dried herbs and adjust the proportions by using about half by volume.

Avocado Dip

Net Carb Count: 4 grams

Ingredients

Avocados	2 (pitted and peeled)
Lemon juice	2 Tbsp
Salt and pepper	to taste
Garlic, minced	2 cloves, roasted

Method

Blend all the ingredients together till you reach the right consistency. Add chopped parsley if you want to vary the flavour a bit.

Desserts
Peanut Butter Cups

Net Carb Count per Cup: 3.6 grams

Ingredients

Butter (unsalted is better)	1 stick
Chocolate, dark, unsweetened	1 ounce
Stevia extract	to taste – add by the drop
Peanut butter	4 Tbsp
Heavy cream	2 Tbsp
Almonds, chopped	16

Method

- Melt the chocolate and butter, either in a double boiler or in the microwave. Mix well, then add the stevia.

- Add the peanut butter and cream. Taste again, and check if you'd like it to be sweeter.

- Line an 8-cup muffin tray with liners and distribute evenly. Freeze.

- Store them in the freezer – they do not stand up to heat at all.

Almond Lemon Cakes

Net Carb Count per cake: 1 gram

Ingredients

Almond flour	¼ cup
Coconut flour	2 Tbsp
Butter	¼ cup
Eggs, whole	3
Coconut milk	1 Tbsp
Lemon juice	1 Tbsp
Erythritol	¼ cup
Baking soda	½ tsp
Vinegar	¼ tsp
Cinnamon	1 tsp
Extract of preference	1 tsp
Liquid stevia	¼ tsp
Salt	1 pinch

Method

- Preheat the oven to 325 degrees Fahrenheit.

- Sieve and mix together the dry ingredients – coconut flour, almond flour, cinnamon, baking soda and salt – together well.

- In another bowl, whisk together eggs, Erythritol, flavouring extract, lemon juice, coconut milk, vinegar, stevia and melted butter till fluffy.

- Add the dry ingredients slowly to the wet ingredients, whisking gently but thoroughly.

- Distribute evenly in your muffin tray and bake for about 16 minutes, or till done. Let it cool before serving.

Spiced Cake in a Mug

Net Carb Count (per serving): 4 grams

Ingredients

Egg, whole	1
Butter	2 Tbsp
Almond flour	2 Tbsp
Erythritol	1 Tbsp
Stevia	a few drops, to taste
Seasoning (cinnamon, clove, ginger)	¼ tsp each
Vanilla extract	¼ tsp

Method:

- Whisk all the ingredients together and microwave in a mug for about 60-70 seconds.

- Let it cool a bit, then turn upside down and thump.

- Serve with whipped heavy cream, if you prefer it so.

Keto Fudge (serves 8 reasonable people)

Net Carb Count (per serving): 1.8 grams

Ingredients

Butter	2 Tbsp
Heavy cream	3 Tbsp
Cream cheese	4 ounces
Liquid stevia	a few drops, to taste
Cocoa powder (unsweetened)	2 Tbsp
Salt	1 pinch

Method

- In a small saucepan, melt the butter. Then add heavy cream, and cream cheese, whisking until you get a nice, smooth consistency.

- Add the sweetener. Taste and adjust.

- Lower the heat till it's simmering gently and add the cocoa and salt. Make sure it's all blended well.

- Transfer to a buttered serving dish and refrigerate very well. Cut into 8 pieces when it's cool and still setting.

Note: This fudge tends to melt very quickly, so keep refrigerated.

Keto Caffeine Blast

Net Carbs – 1 gram

Ingredients

Coffee	1 cup
Butter, unsalted	1 Tbsp
Coconut oil	1 Tbsp
Heavy cream	1 Tbsp
Vanilla extract	1 tsp
Cinnamon	¼ tsp

Method:

- Brew coffee as you usually do. Into a cup of hot coffee, add the butter and the coconut oil, then the cream.

- Season, add liquid stevia if you need a sweetener. Mix it all very well.

- You'll be having this a lot, so experiment with all the flavours you can think of.

Chocolate Shake

Net Carb Count : 6.7 grams

Ingredients

Coconut milk	1 cup 4
Heavy cream	½ cup
Liquid stevia	to taste
Ice	1 cup
Cocoa powder, unsweetened	1 Tbsp

Method

Chuck everything in the blender and blitz. That's it! Quick meal.

Avocado-coconut smoothie

Net Carb Count: 6.3 grams

Ingredients

Coconut milk	1 Cup
Avocado	1
Cocoa powder	1 Tbsp
Butter	1 Tbsp
Ice cubes	To your preference

Method:

Blend everything together. Add a few drops of stevia if you'd like it sweeter.

Conclusion

I sincerely hope that you have enjoyed this book and that it starts you on a path of health and wellness. It is my desire that my readers become extremely successful in completing this healthier lifestyle. Again, thanks so much for reading.

www.ingramcontent.com/pod-product-compliance
Lightning Source LLC
Chambersburg PA
CBHW070303290526
45791CB00003B/1068